# Dealing with Lichen Sclerosus

## Management and Self Care of Lichen Sclerosus

By

Bart Rayan

Copyright@2023

# Table of Contents

# CHAPTER 1

# LICHEN SCLEROSUS

Lichen sclerosus (LS) is a chronic inflammatory skin condition that primarily affects the genital and anogenital regions, but can also involve other areas of the body. It is more common in women, although it can occur in men and children as well. LS causes thinning, whitening, and atrophy of the skin, leading to various symptoms and potential complications.

The exact cause of lichen sclerosus is unknown, but it is

believed to involve a combination of genetic predisposition, autoimmune factors, and hormonal imbalances. It is not contagious and cannot be transmitted through sexual or other forms of contact.

Symptoms of lichen sclerosus can vary between individuals but commonly include intense itching, discomfort, and pain in the affected areas. In women, the condition often affects the vulva, causing white, patchy skin and adhesions that may lead to pain during sexual intercourse. In men, LS can involve the foreskin, causing tightness, difficulty retracting the foreskin, and urinary problems. Both men and women can experience LS affecting the anus and perianal area, resulting in itching, discomfort, and painful bowel movements.

The treatment of lichen sclerosus aims to relieve symptoms, prevent complications, and improve the quality of life for affected individuals. The primary approach involves the use of topical corticosteroids, which help reduce inflammation and alleviate symptoms. Calcineurin inhibitors and retinoids may also be prescribed in certain cases. Additionally, self-care measures such as maintaining good hygiene practices, using moisturizers, and avoiding irritants can help manage symptoms.

If lichen sclerosus leads to scarring and fusion of the genital tissues, surgical interventions may be necessary to release adhesions and restore functionality. Regular follow-up care and monitoring are important to detect any potential complications, such as secondary infections or the rare development of squamous cell carcinoma.

Living with lichen sclerosus can have a significant impact on a person's physical and emotional well-being. The condition can cause distress, affect self-esteem, and interfere with sexual functioning. Therefore, support from healthcare professionals, psychological counseling, and support groups can be beneficial in managing the emotional and psychological aspects of living with LS.

While there is no known cure for lichen sclerosus, the condition can often be effectively managed with appropriate treatment and lifestyle modifications. With ongoing research and advancements in understanding the underlying mechanisms, there is hope for improved treatment options and a better prognosis for individuals with lichen sclerosus in the future.

It is important to consult with a healthcare professional for an accurate diagnosis and personalized treatment plan if you suspect you may have lichen sclerosus or are experiencing any concerning symptoms.

## Complications and long-term effects:

If left untreated or poorly managed, lichen sclerosus can lead to various complications and long-term effects. Scarring and atrophy of the affected skin are common outcomes, which can result in functional impairment and deformity. The scarring may cause the labia to shrink or fuse together, leading to a narrowing of the vaginal opening, which can make sexual intercourse difficult or painful. In severe cases, scarring can cause urinary obstruction or strictures in the urethra. Additionally, the affected skin becomes more vulnerable to secondary infections, such as bacterial or fungal infections, which can further exacerbate symptoms and complicate the treatment process. Long-standing lichen sclerosus also carries a slightly increased risk of developing squamous cell carcinoma, a type of skin cancer, although this risk is generally low.

**Living with lichen sclerosus:**
Lichen sclerosus can have a significant impact on an individual's daily life and emotional well-being. The chronic nature of the condition, coupled with the potential for discomfort, pain, and interference with sexual function, can lead to frustration, embarrassment, and anxiety. It is essential for individuals with lichen sclerosus to seek emotional support and education about the condition. This may involve counseling, joining support groups, or accessing online resources that provide information and a platform for sharing experiences with others

facing similar challenges. Additionally, adopting self-care practices, such as maintaining good hygiene, using appropriate moisturizers and emollients, and avoiding irritants, can help alleviate symptoms and improve overall well-being.

**Prevention and outlook:**

While the exact cause of lichen sclerosus remains unknown, there are no known definitive strategies for preventing its development. However, early diagnosis, prompt treatment, and diligent management can help minimize symptoms, prevent complications, and improve the long-term outlook for individuals with lichen sclerosus. Regular follow-up appointments with healthcare professionals are important for monitoring the condition, assessing treatment effectiveness, and detecting any potential complications or disease progression.

Research and future directions: Lichen sclerosus is an area of ongoing research, and scientists are working to better understand its underlying mechanisms and improve treatment options. Current research efforts focus on investigating the role of genetic factors, immune dysregulation, and hormonal influences in the development and progression of lichen sclerosus. Researchers are also exploring potential novel therapies and targeted treatments to enhance symptom control and prevent long-term complications. Continued research and advancements in the field hold promise for improved diagnostic tools, more effective treatment strategies, and ultimately, a better quality of life for individuals affected by lichen sclerosus.

Lichen sclerosus is a chronic inflammatory skin condition primarily affecting the genital and anogenital regions. It can cause significant discomfort, pain, and emotional distress if not properly managed. Timely diagnosis, appropriate treatment, and diligent self-care practices can help individuals with lichen sclerosus achieve symptom relief and prevent complications. Seeking support from healthcare professionals, counseling, and support groups can also be valuable in managing the psychological and emotional aspects of living with this condition. With ongoing research and advancements, the outlook for individuals with lichen sclerosus continues to improve, offering hope for better treatment options and an improved quality of life in the future.

# CHAPTER 2

## SYMPTOMS AND CLINICAL PRESENTATION

### Genital Symptoms

Genital symptoms are common in lichen sclerosus (LS) and can significantly impact the quality of life for individuals affected by the condition. LS primarily affects the genital region, including the vulva in women and the foreskin and glans penis in men. The following are the genital symptoms associated with LS.

## Itching and Discomfort

One of the hallmark symptoms of lichen sclerosus is intense itching (pruritus) in the genital area. The itching can be persistent, bothersome, and interfere with daily activities, sleep, and overall well-being. It may worsen at night or during periods of increased warmth or humidity. The exact cause of the itching is not fully understood, but it is believed to be related to the inflammatory processes and changes in the affected skin.

The itchiness in lichen sclerosus can be severe and relentless, leading to constant scratching and subsequent skin damage.

Excessive scratching can further irritate the skin, cause excoriation (skin erosion), and increase the risk of developing secondary infections. The continuous itch-scratch cycle can create a significant burden for individuals with lichen sclerosus, affecting their physical comfort and psychological state.

## Painful Intercourse

Painful intercourse, also known as dyspareunia, is a distressing symptom experienced by many women with lichen sclerosus. The inflammation and thinning of the vulvar tissues can result in decreased elasticity, dryness, and fragility, making sexual intercourse uncomfortable or even excruciatingly painful. The pain may be described as a burning, stinging, or tearing sensation, and it can persist for hours or even days after sexual activity.

The fear and anticipation of pain during intercourse can lead to anxiety, decreased libido, and strain on intimate relationships. As a result, individuals with lichen sclerosus may experience sexual dysfunction, reduced sexual satisfaction, and a decreased overall quality of life.

## White, Patchy Skin

Another characteristic genital symptom of lichen sclerosus is the presence of white, patchy skin in the affected area. The affected skin may appear thin, fragile, and crinkled, resembling parchment or cigarette paper. This phenomenon is commonly referred to as "cigarette paper" or "candyfloss" skin.

The white, patchy areas in lichen sclerosus are often accompanied by loss of skin elasticity and atrophy. The affected skin may feel tight, restricting movement and causing discomfort. The whitened areas may extend beyond the visible borders and may involve the labia majora, labia minora, clitoral hood, perianal region, and even extend to the inner thighs.

In some cases, lichen sclerosus can cause the labia minora to shrink or fuse together, resulting in a narrowing of the vaginal opening. This condition, known as labial adhesion or labial fusion, can further contribute to pain during sexual intercourse, urinary difficulties, and challenges with menstrual hygiene.

The white, patchy skin in lichen sclerosus is a result of the underlying inflammation and disruption of normal skin structure. The loss of pigmentation is due to the destruction of melanocytes, the cells responsible for producing skin pigment. The affected areas may be more prone to bruising, bleeding, and the formation of skin tears (fissures).

It is important to note that lichen sclerosus can affect the genital region differently in men. In males, LS commonly involves the foreskin (prepuce) and the glans penis. The symptoms may include itching, discomfort, tightening of the foreskin (phimosis), and difficulty retracting the foreskin (paraphimosis).

The genital symptoms of lichen sclerosus encompass intense itching and discomfort, painful intercourse, and the presence of white, patchy skin. These symptoms can have a significant impact on an individual's physical comfort, sexual function, and overall quality of life. Seeking prompt medical evaluation and appropriate treatment can help alleviate these symptoms and improve well-being.

## Extragenital Symptoms

While lichen sclerosus (LS) primarily affects the genital region, it can also involve extragenital areas of the body. The condition may extend beyond the genital region to affect the skin around the anus, perianal area, and other non-genital areas. The following are the extragenital symptoms associated with LS.

## Anus and Perianal Area

Lichen sclerosus can affect the skin around the anus and the perianal area, leading to a range of symptoms and complications. These symptoms can be similar to those experienced in the genital region, but the presentation may vary.

Itching and discomfort: Individuals with lichen sclerosus in the anus and perianal area often experience itching (pruritus) and discomfort. The itching can be intense and persistent, causing significant distress. It may be accompanied by a constant urge to scratch, leading to further irritation and potential skin damage. The discomfort can range from a mild irritation to a more severe burning or stinging sensation.

Pain and fissures: LS in the anus and perianal area can cause pain, especially during bowel movements. The skin may become fragile and prone to developing small tears or fissures. These fissures can be painful and may cause bleeding. The presence of fissures can further contribute to discomfort and may make bowel movements a painful and distressing experience.

Difficulty with hygiene: Lichen sclerosus affecting the perianal area can make hygiene practices challenging. The inflammation and thinning of the affected skin can make cleaning the area difficult, leading to potential hygiene-related issues and discomfort. It is important to maintain good hygiene practices while being gentle to avoid further irritation or injury to the affected skin.

## Other Affected Areas

In addition to the genital and perianal regions, lichen sclerosus can occasionally involve other areas of the body, although it is less common. The non-genital areas that may be affected include the breasts, upper body, lower body, and extremities.

Breasts: Lichen sclerosus can affect the skin on the breasts, particularly the areolas and nipples. The affected skin may become thin, atrophic, and white in appearance. Itching, discomfort, and pain may also be present. In severe cases, scarring and distortion of the breast shape can occur.

Upper body: LS can manifest on the upper body, including the neck, shoulders, and upper arms, although this occurrence is relatively rare. The symptoms in these areas are similar to those seen in the genital region, including itching, discomfort, and white, patchy skin.

Lower body and extremities: Lichen sclerosus can occasionally affect the skin on the lower body, such as the thighs and buttocks. The symptoms in these areas are similar to those seen in the genital region, including itching, discomfort, and the presence of white, patchy skin. In some cases, LS may extend to involve the skin on the lower legs and feet.

It is important to note that while lichen sclerosus can affect these extragenital areas, the severity and frequency of involvement can vary between individuals. In some cases, lichen sclerosus may solely affect the genital region without involvement of extragenital areas.

Managing Extragenital Symptoms: The management of extragenital symptoms in lichen sclerosus involves similar approaches to those used for genital symptoms. Topical corticosteroids are often prescribed to reduce inflammation and relieve symptoms. Emollients and moisturizers may be recommended to soothe and hydrate the affected skin. It is important to follow proper hygiene practices and avoid irritants that may worsen symptoms. If there are complications such as fissures or infections, additional medical interventions may be necessary, including the use of antibiotics or other specific treatments.

lichen sclerosus can extend beyond the genital region to involve extragenital areas such as the anus, perianal region, breasts, and other non-genital regions. Symptoms in these areas may include itching, discomfort, pain, and the presence of white, patchy skin. Proper management, including appropriate topical treatments and hygiene practices, can help alleviate symptoms and improve the overall well-being of individuals with lichen sclerosus.

# CHAPTER 3

# MANAGEMENT AND SELF-CARE

## Hygiene Practices

Maintaining good hygiene practices is essential for managing lichen sclerosus (LS) and minimizing symptoms. Proper hygiene can help keep the affected skin clean, reduce the risk of infections, and promote overall comfort. The following are some key hygiene practices that individuals with LS should consider:

Gentle cleansing: When cleaning the affected area, it is important to use gentle and non-irritating products. Avoid using harsh soaps, perfumed cleansers, or products that contain potential irritants such as alcohol or fragrances. Instead, opt for mild, unscented cleansers or emollient washes that are specifically formulated for sensitive skin. Gently cleanse the area with lukewarm water, using your hand or a soft cloth, and pat dry with a soft towel.

Avoid irritants: It is important to avoid potential irritants that can worsen LS symptoms or cause further inflammation. This includes avoiding harsh detergents, fabric softeners, scented toilet paper, and tight-fitting synthetic underwear. Opt for loose-fitting cotton underwear and clothing to allow for better air circulation and minimize friction.

Avoid excessive moisture: Excessive moisture in the affected area can exacerbate symptoms and increase the risk of secondary infections. After cleansing, make sure to thoroughly dry the area, paying attention to any skin folds. Use a clean, soft towel and gently pat dry, avoiding rubbing or friction. It may be helpful to use a separate towel specifically for the affected area to prevent the spread of potential infections.

Appropriate menstrual hygiene: For women with LS, managing menstrual hygiene is important. It is recommended to use unscented, hypoallergenic menstrual products, such as pads or tampons, to minimize irritation. Changing these products frequently is important to maintain cleanliness and prevent prolonged exposure to moisture.

After toileting practices: After using the toilet, it is advisable to gently cleanse the affected area with lukewarm water and pat dry. Avoid using rough toilet paper or wipes that may contain irritants or fragrances. Some individuals find it helpful to use a peri-bottle or a gentle cleansing spray to maintain hygiene without causing further irritation.

Regular follow-up appointments: Regular follow-up appointments with healthcare professionals are essential for monitoring the condition, assessing treatment effectiveness, and detecting any potential complications or disease progression. These appointments provide an opportunity to discuss any concerns, receive guidance on self-care practices, and make necessary adjustments to the treatment plan.

# Moisturizers and Emollients

Moisturizers and emollients play a crucial role in managing lichen sclerosus by hydrating and protecting the affected skin. They help alleviate dryness, reduce itching, and improve overall comfort. The following are key considerations when using moisturizers and emollients:

Choose the right product: Selecting an appropriate moisturizer or emollient is important. Look for products that are fragrance-free, hypoallergenic, and specifically formulated for sensitive skin. opt for thicker ointments or creams rather than lotions, as they provide better hydration and protection. Ingredients such as petrolatum, shea butter, cocoa butter, or ceramides are commonly found in moisturizers and can be beneficial for maintaining skin hydration.

Application technique: Apply moisturizers or emollients to the affected area after cleansing and drying. Take a small amount of the product and gently massage it into the skin using circular motions. Ensure thorough coverage of the affected areas, including the vulva, perianal region, or any other areas affected by LS. Avoid excessive rubbing or pressure that may further irritate the skin.

Frequency of application: The frequency of moisturizer application may vary depending on individual needs and the severity of symptoms. In general, it is recommended to apply moisturizers at least twice a day or as directed by a healthcare professional. However, some individuals may require more frequent application, especially during periods of increased dryness or itching. Listen to your body and adjust the frequency of application as needed.

Timing of application: Applying moisturizers or emollients at specific times can be beneficial. For instance, applying them after bathing or showering when the skin is still slightly damp can help lock in moisture and enhance absorption. Additionally, applying moisturizers before bedtime can provide overnight hydration and relieve symptoms that may worsen during sleep.

Combining with other treatments: Moisturizers and emollients can be used in combination with other prescribed treatments for lichen sclerosus, such as topical corticosteroids. Follow the instructions provided by your healthcare professional and ensure proper spacing between the application of different products to allow each one to be effectively absorbed.

Patch testing: Some individuals with LS may have sensitivities or allergies to certain ingredients found in moisturizers or emollients. If you suspect a reaction to a product, perform a patch test before applying it to larger areas. Apply a small amount of the product to a small, discreet area of skin and monitor for any adverse reactions such as redness, itching, or irritation. If a reaction occurs, discontinue use and consult with a healthcare professional.

practicing good hygiene, including gentle cleansing and avoiding irritants, is crucial in managing lichen sclerosus. Incorporating moisturizers and emollients into the daily routine can provide hydration, relieve dryness, and improve overall comfort. It is important to choose suitable products, follow proper application techniques, and seek guidance from healthcare professionals for personalized advice on managing the condition effectively.

## Lifestyle Modifications

In addition to medical treatments, certain lifestyle modifications can help manage lichen sclerosus

(LS) and reduce the frequency and severity of symptoms. Making positive changes in daily habits and routines can contribute to overall well-being and minimize triggers that may exacerbate LS symptoms. The following are some lifestyle modifications that individuals with LS may consider:

Stress management: Stress can have a significant impact on the immune system and may trigger or worsen LS symptoms. Finding effective stress management techniques, such as relaxation exercises, meditation, deep breathing, or engaging in hobbies or activities that bring joy and relaxation, can be beneficial.

Incorporating stress reduction practices into daily life can help minimize LS flare-ups and improve overall quality of life.

Avoiding irritants: Identify and avoid potential irritants that may worsen LS symptoms or trigger flare-ups. This includes avoiding harsh soaps, perfumed detergents, scented products, and tight-fitting clothing made of synthetic materials. opt for gentle, unscented products and clothing made from breathable fabrics such as cotton.

Avoiding excessive heat and moisture: Excessive heat and moisture can exacerbate LS symptoms and increase discomfort. Avoid prolonged exposure to hot baths, saunas, or hot tubs, as well as tight occlusive clothing that may trap heat and moisture. opt for loose-fitting, breathable clothing and avoid activities that may lead to excessive sweating in the genital area.

Maintaining a healthy weight: Obesity and excess weight can contribute to inflammation and exacerbate LS symptoms. Maintaining a healthy weight through a balanced diet and regular exercise can help manage LS and improve overall well-being. Consult with a healthcare professional or registered dietitian for personalized advice on nutrition and weight management.

Avoiding tobacco and alcohol: Tobacco and alcohol consumption can have detrimental effects on the immune system and overall health. These substances may worsen LS symptoms and increase the risk of complications. It is advisable to refrain from smoking and limit alcohol intake to promote optimal health and LS management.

Proper wound care: Individuals with LS may be prone to skin tears, fissures, or open sores in the affected areas. It is important to practice proper wound care to prevent infection and promote healing. Cleanse the area gently with mild soap and lukewarm water, apply appropriate wound care products as recommended by a healthcare professional, and cover the wound with a sterile dressing if necessary. Seek medical attention for any signs of infection or non-healing wounds.

## Follow-up Care and Monitoring

Regular follow-up care and monitoring are crucial for individuals with lichen sclerosus. These aspects ensure that the condition is appropriately managed, symptoms are controlled, and any potential complications are detected and addressed in a timely manner. The following are key considerations regarding follow-up care and monitoring:

Scheduled follow-up appointments: It is important to attend scheduled follow-up appointments with a healthcare professional who specializes in dermatology or gynecology, depending on the affected area. These appointments allow for regular assessment of the condition, evaluation of treatment effectiveness, and adjustment of the management plan as needed. They also provide an opportunity to discuss any concerns or questions and receive guidance on self-care practices.

Monitoring for disease progression: Lichen sclerosus has the potential to progress over time, leading to complications such as scarring, fusion of the labia, or functional impairments. Regular monitoring allows healthcare professionals to detect any signs of disease progression and intervene accordingly. This may involve visual examinations, biopsies, or other diagnostic tests to evaluate the extent of the condition and guide treatment decisions.

Routine self-examinations: Individuals with lichen sclerosus can also play an active role in monitoring their own condition. Perform routine self-examinations to observe any changes in the affected areas. Look for signs of worsening symptoms, such as increased redness, itching, or changes in skin texture. Promptly report any concerning findings to a healthcare professional for further evaluation and management.

Education and support: Seek educational resources and support groups dedicated to lichen sclerosus. Understanding the condition, its potential complications, and available management options can empower individuals to actively participate in their own care. Support groups provide an opportunity to connect with others who are facing similar challenges, share experiences, and exchange information and support.

It is important to remember that lichen sclerosus is a chronic condition that requires ongoing management. By implementing lifestyle modifications, attending regular follow-up appointments, and actively monitoring the condition, individuals with LS can optimize their treatment outcomes, improve their quality of life, and effectively manage the symptoms associated with the condition.

# CHAPTER 4

# COMPLICATIONS AND LONG-TERM EFFECTS

## Scarring and Atrophy

One of the most significant complications of lichen sclerosus is the potential for scarring and atrophy in the affected areas. Scarring refers to the formation of fibrous tissue, which can lead to the tightening and loss of elasticity in the skin. Atrophy refers to the thinning of the skin, making it more fragile and susceptible to injury. Scarring and atrophy can have various implications for individuals with LS:

Functional impairment: The scarring and atrophy caused by LS can result in functional impairments. In the genital area, the narrowing and fusion of the labia or clitoral hood can cause discomfort, pain, and difficulties with urination or sexual intercourse. In some cases, scarring may also lead to the closure of the vaginal opening, resulting in a condition known as introital stenosis. These functional impairments can significantly impact the quality of life and well-being of individuals with LS.

Aesthetic concerns: Scarring and atrophy can cause visible changes in the affected areas, leading to aesthetic concerns. The skin may appear pale, thin, wrinkled, or have a parchment-like texture. These changes can be distressing for individuals, affecting body image and self-esteem.

Increased risk of trauma: The fragile and thin skin associated with LS is more susceptible to trauma and injury. Even minor friction or trauma to the affected areas can lead to tears, fissures, or open sores. These wounds can be painful, slow to heal, and prone to infection. Proper wound care and cautious management of the affected areas are crucial to minimize the risk of trauma-related complications.

## Secondary Infections

Lichen sclerosus can also increase the susceptibility to secondary infections in the affected areas. The compromised skin barrier, inflammation, and itching associated with LS create an environment conducive to the growth of bacteria, fungi, and other microorganisms. Common types of infections that may occur in individuals with LS include:

Bacterial infections: The damaged skin in LS can become colonized by bacteria, leading to infections such as cellulitis or abscesses. Symptoms of bacterial infections may include redness, warmth, swelling, pain, and the presence of pus. Prompt medical attention and appropriate antibiotic treatment are essential to manage bacterial infections effectively and prevent their spread.

Fungal infections: Fungal infections, such as candidiasis (yeast infection), are also more common in individuals with LS. The warm and moist environment created by LS can promote the overgrowth of yeast or other fungi. Symptoms of fungal infections may include itching, redness, soreness, and a cottage cheese-like discharge. Antifungal medications, either topical or oral, are typically prescribed to treat fungal infections.

Viral infections: While less common, viral infections can also occur in individuals with LS. Herpes simplex virus (HSV) infections, for example, may manifest as painful blisters or sores in the affected areas. Antiviral medications may be prescribed to manage viral infections and reduce symptoms.

Preventing secondary infections is an important aspect of managing lichen sclerosus. Practicing good hygiene, avoiding irritants, and keeping the affected areas clean and dry can help reduce the risk of infections. It is also crucial to promptly address any signs of infection, such as increased redness, swelling, pain, or discharge, and seek appropriate medical treatment.

## Sexual Dysfunction

Lichen sclerosus (LS) can have a significant impact on sexual function and intimacy for both men and women. The symptoms and complications associated with LS can contribute to sexual dysfunction in various ways:

Painful intercourse (dyspareunia): One of the most common sexual complaints in individuals with LS is painful intercourse. The scarring, atrophy, and inflammation of the genital area can make sexual activity uncomfortable or even unbearable. Pain during intercourse can result in decreased sexual desire, avoidance of sexual activity, and strained intimate relationships.

Reduced sexual desire (hypolibidemia): LS can also lead to a decreased sexual desire or libido. The physical discomfort, emotional distress, and body image concerns associated with LS may contribute to a diminished interest in sexual activity. Additionally, the impact of LS on body image and self-esteem can affect sexual confidence and desire.

Difficulty with arousal and orgasm: LS may interfere with the normal physiological responses of arousal and orgasm. The discomfort, pain, or physical limitations caused by LS can make it challenging to achieve or maintain arousal. Furthermore, the emotional stress and anxiety associated with LS can further disrupt sexual response and orgasmic function.

Psychological impact: The impact of LS on sexual function extends beyond the physical symptoms. The chronic nature of the condition, its impact on body image, and the challenges it presents to sexual intimacy can lead to psychological distress, anxiety, and depression. These psychological factors can further contribute to sexual dysfunction.

It is essential for individuals with LS to communicate openly with their healthcare professionals about any sexual concerns or difficulties they may be experiencing. There are various strategies and treatment options available to manage sexual dysfunction associated with LS, including:

Topical therapies: Topical corticosteroids or other immunomodulatory medications prescribed for LS can help reduce inflammation, alleviate symptoms, and improve sexual comfort. Applying these medications as directed by a healthcare professional may help reduce pain and discomfort during intercourse.

Sexual counseling: Seeking support from a qualified sexual counselor or therapist who specializes in working with individuals with chronic conditions can be beneficial.

These professionals can provide guidance, support, and practical strategies to address sexual concerns, enhance communication with partners, and improve overall sexual well-being.

Lifestyle modifications: Implementing lifestyle modifications, such as stress reduction techniques, relaxation exercises, and open communication with partners, can help alleviate sexual difficulties associated with LS. Reducing stress and creating a supportive and understanding sexual environment can positively impact sexual function and intimacy.

Emotional support: Dealing with the challenges of LS and sexual dysfunction can be emotionally challenging. Seeking emotional support from loved ones, support groups, or counseling services can help individuals cope with the psychological impact of LS and improve overall well-being.

It is important to remember that sexual dysfunction associated with LS is a valid concern, and individuals should not hesitate to seek help and support. By working with healthcare professionals and addressing sexual concerns, individuals with LS can explore strategies to enhance sexual comfort, improve intimacy, and maintain a satisfying sexual relationship.

# Squamous Cell Carcinoma

While rare, a potential long-term complication of lichen sclerosus (LS) is the development of squamous cell carcinoma (SCC). SCC is a type of skin cancer that can occur in the areas affected by LS, particularly the genital region. It is important to understand the risk factors, signs, and management of SCC in individuals with LS:

Risk factors: The exact cause of SCC development in LS is not fully understood. However, long-standing and severe cases of LS, particularly those that have not been appropriately treated or managed, are believed to have a higher risk of progressing to SCC. Other potential risk factors include male gender, tobacco use, and a history of other skin cancers.

Signs and symptoms: The development of SCC in LS can present with various signs and symptoms. These may include persistent ulcers or sores that do not heal, thickened or raised areas of skin, changes in skin color or texture, bleeding or crusting, and the presence of a lump or mass. Any suspicious skin changes or lesions should be promptly evaluated by a healthcare professional.

Monitoring and surveillance: Regular monitoring and surveillance are crucial in individuals with LS to detect early signs of SCC. This typically involves routine clinical examinations and potentially additional tests, such as biopsies or imaging studies, to assess the affected areas and identify any suspicious changes. The frequency and extent of surveillance may vary based on individual risk factors and the severity of LS.

Treatment: If SCC is detected in individuals with LS, prompt treatment is necessary. The treatment options for SCC depend on the stage and extent of the cancer. These may include surgical excision, radiation therapy, chemotherapy, or a combination of these approaches. Early detection and intervention can improve treatment outcomes and prognosis.

Prevention: While the development of SCC in LS cannot always be prevented, there are measures individuals can take to minimize the risk. This includes diligent management of LS symptoms, regular follow-up care, and adherence to treatment plans recommended by healthcare professionals. It is important to report any concerning changes or symptoms promptly to ensure timely evaluation and intervention.

It is essential for individuals with LS to remain vigilant and proactive in monitoring their condition and seeking appropriate medical attention. Routine follow-up care, adherence to treatment plans, and prompt reporting of any concerning skin changes are crucial to detect and manage SCC at its earliest stages.

Overall, while the development of SCC in LS is relatively rare, it highlights the importance of long-term management, surveillance, and proactive healthcare involvement. By staying informed, practicing good self-care, and working closely with healthcare professionals, individuals with LS can minimize the risk of complications and maintain optimal health.

## Long-term Effects and Prognosis

The long-term effects and prognosis of lichen sclerosus can vary among individuals. Some individuals may experience relatively mild symptoms and minimal complications, while others may face more significant challenges. The following are important considerations regarding the long-term effects and prognosis of LS:

Chronic nature: Lichen sclerosus is a chronic condition, which means that it typically persists over a lifetime. While symptoms may come and go or vary in intensity, ongoing management and monitoring are necessary to ensure optimal outcomes and minimize complications.

Progression of the condition: Lichen sclerosus can progress over time, leading to increased symptoms and the potential for complications. Regular follow-up appointments and monitoring allow healthcare professionals to assess disease progression and adjust treatment plans accordingly. Not all individuals with LS will experience disease progression, but it is important to remain vigilant and address any changes or worsening of symptoms promptly.

Effectiveness of treatment: With appropriate management and treatment, the symptoms of lichen sclerosus can often be effectively controlled. Topical corticosteroids, the mainstay of treatment, can help reduce inflammation and alleviate symptoms. Other treatment options, such as calcineurin inhibitors, may be considered in cases where corticosteroids are not effective or well-tolerated. However, it is important to note that the response to treatment can vary among individuals, and finding the most suitable approach may require some trial and error.

Regular monitoring: Regular follow-up care and monitoring are crucial for individuals with lichen sclerosus. This allows healthcare professionals to assess treatment efficacy, monitor for disease progression or complications, and provide guidance on self-care practices. Follow-up appointments also provide an opportunity to address any concerns, discuss changes in symptoms, and make necessary adjustments to the treatment plan.

while lichen sclerosus can pose challenges and potential complications, with appropriate management, individuals can effectively control symptoms and minimize long-term effects. Collaborating with healthcare professionals, adhering to treatment plans, and implementing self-care strategies are essential for optimizing outcomes and improving quality of life for individuals with lichen sclerosus.

# CHAPTER 5

# PREVENTION AND OUTLOOK

## Prevention Strategies

While the exact cause of lichen sclerosus (LS) remains unknown, there are certain strategies that may help reduce the risk of developing the condition or minimize its severity. Although not all cases of LS can be prevented, adopting healthy habits and implementing preventive measures can be beneficial. some prevention strategies that may be considered:

1. Maintain good hygiene: Practicing good hygiene is important in preventing various skin conditions, including LS. Keep the genital area clean and dry, and avoid using harsh soaps or irritating substances that can disrupt the natural balance of the skin.

2. Wear loose-fitting clothing: Wearing loose-fitting clothing made from breathable fabrics, such as cotton, can help minimize friction and promote airflow, reducing the risk of irritation and moisture buildup in the genital area.

3. Avoid potential irritants: Avoid using products that may irritate the genital area, such as perfumed soaps, bubble baths, and feminine hygiene sprays. These products can disrupt the natural pH balance of the skin and increase the risk of irritation.

4. Manage underlying conditions: LS has been associated with certain autoimmune disorders, such as thyroid diseases and vitiligo. Managing these underlying conditions through regular medical care and appropriate

treatment may help reduce the risk or severity of LS.

5. Regular self-examinations: Performing regular self-examinations of the genital area can help detect any changes or early signs of LS. If any unusual symptoms or skin changes are noticed, seeking medical attention promptly can facilitate early diagnosis and treatment.

6. Routine follow-up care: If diagnosed with LS, it is essential to adhere to routine follow-up care and monitoring as recommended by a

healthcare professional. Regular check-ups can help detect any recurrence, manage symptoms, and address any potential complications.

While these preventive measures may help reduce the risk or severity of LS, it is important to note that the condition can still develop despite taking preventive steps. LS is a complex disorder with various underlying factors, and its development is not entirely preventable.

# Prognosis and Long-Term Outlook

The prognosis for individuals with lichen sclerosus (LS) varies depending on several factors, including the severity of the condition, response to treatment, and individual characteristics.

1. Disease progression: LS is a chronic condition that tends to progress slowly over time. The disease course is highly variable, and its progression can be unpredictable. Some individuals may experience periods of remission or stabilization, while others may have persistent or

recurrent symptoms. Regular medical care and adherence to treatment can help manage the symptoms and minimize disease progression.

2. Treatment response: The response to treatment varies among individuals with LS. With appropriate medical interventions, many people experience improvement in symptoms and quality of life. However, complete resolution of LS may not always be achievable. It is important to work closely with a healthcare professional to find the most effective treatment

regimen and to monitor and adjust the treatment as needed.

3. Complications and long-term effects: LS can lead to various complications, including scarring, atrophy, secondary infections, and sexual dysfunction. These complications can significantly impact an individual's quality of life. Timely diagnosis, proper management, and regular follow-up care can help prevent or minimize the occurrence of complications and long-term effects.

4. Risk of malignancy: There is a small but increased risk of developing squamous cell carcinoma (SCC) in the affected areas of LS. Regular monitoring and surveillance are essential to detect any suspicious changes or early signs of malignancy. With proper medical care and timely intervention, the risk of developing SCC can be effectively managed.

5. Psychological impact: Living with a chronic condition like LS can have a psychological impact on individuals. It may affect body image, self-esteem,

and sexual well-being. Seeking psychological support, such as counseling or support groups, can be beneficial in managing the emotional and psychological aspects of LS and improving overall well-being.

It is important to remember that LS is a chronic condition that requires ongoing management and monitoring. Adhering to a treatment plan, practicing self-care measures, and maintaining regular follow-up care are crucial for long-term disease control and symptom management. While LS can have significant physical and emotional impacts, with appropriate care and support, many individuals can effectively manage the condition and lead fulfilling lives.

while it is not possible to completely prevent lichen sclerosus, adopting good hygiene practices, wearing loose-fitting clothing, avoiding potential irritants, managing underlying conditions, performing regular self-examinations, and seeking routine follow-up care can help reduce the risk or severity of the condition. The long-term outlook for individuals with LS varies depending on the individual's response to treatment, disease progression, occurrence of complications, and overall management of the condition. With proper medical care, lifestyle modifications, and psychological support, many individuals with LS can effectively manage the condition and maintain a good quality of life.

# CHAPTER 6

# IMPACT ON QUALITY OF LIFE AND PSYCHOLOGICAL WELL-BEING

## Body Image and Self-esteem

Lichen sclerosus (LS) can have a significant impact on the body image and self-esteem of individuals affected by the condition. The visible symptoms and physical changes associated with LS, particularly in the genital area, can cause distress and affect how individuals perceive themselves. Here are the impact of LS on body image and self-esteem and discuss strategies to cope with these challenges.

1. Visible Changes and Discomfort: LS often presents with visible symptoms such as white, patchy skin, scarring, and atrophy in the genital area. These changes can be physically uncomfortable and can also contribute to feelings of self-consciousness and embarrassment. Individuals may experience distress related to the appearance of their genitalia, which can

have a negative impact on body image and self-esteem.

2. Sexual Function and Intimacy: LS can affect sexual function and intimate relationships. Painful intercourse, discomfort, and changes in genital appearance may lead to anxiety, avoidance of sexual activities, and challenges in maintaining intimacy. This can impact self-esteem and create strain in relationships.

3. Social Stigma and Misunderstanding: Due to the intimate nature of LS

symptoms, individuals may feel embarrassed or stigmatized, leading to social isolation and a reluctance to seek support or discuss their condition openly. Lack of awareness and understanding among the general public and even healthcare providers can further contribute to feelings of isolation and low self-esteem.

4. Emotional and Psychological Impact: Living with a chronic condition like LS can take a toll on an individual's emotional well-being. Anxiety, depression,

frustration, and lowered self-confidence are common emotional responses. Dealing with the physical discomfort, ongoing treatment, and uncertainty about the course of the disease can contribute to psychological distress and affect self-esteem.

Coping Strategies:

1. Education and Support: Learning about LS, its symptoms, and treatment options can help individuals feel more empowered and in control of their condition. Support from

healthcare providers, patient advocacy groups, and online communities can provide valuable information, emotional support, and a sense of belonging.

2. Open Communication: Talking openly about LS with trusted friends, family members, or partners can help alleviate feelings of isolation and foster understanding and support. Discussing concerns, fears, and emotional challenges related to LS can help individuals feel heard and validated.

3. Counseling and Therapy: Seeking professional counseling or therapy can be beneficial for addressing the emotional impact of LS. A therapist experienced in working with individuals with chronic conditions can provide strategies to manage anxiety, depression, and body image concerns. Cognitive-behavioral therapy (CBT) may help challenge negative thoughts and improve self-esteem.

4. Self-Care and Body Positivity: Engaging in self-care activities that promote self-acceptance and body

positivity can have a positive impact on body image and self-esteem. This can include practicing mindfulness, engaging in activities that bring joy, and developing a positive relationship with one's body through self-affirmation and self-compassion.

5. Support Groups: Joining support groups specifically tailored to LS can provide a sense of community and a platform to share experiences, coping strategies, and emotional support. Connecting with others who have similar

experiences can be empowering and help individuals realize they are not alone in their journey.

It is important to recognize that addressing the impact of LS on body image and self-esteem is a personal and ongoing process. Different strategies may work for different individuals, and it may take time to find what works best. Seeking professional guidance and support from healthcare providers and mental health professionals can be instrumental in navigating these challenges and promoting overall well-being.

# Coping Strategies and Support

Coping with the challenges of living with lichen sclerosus (LS) can be demanding, both physically and emotionally. Having a supportive network, utilizing coping strategies, and seeking professional assistance can help individuals manage the impact of LS on their quality of life and psychological well-being. These are some coping strategies and available support to navigate the challenges associated with LS.

1. Education and Understanding: Educating oneself about LS and

understanding the condition can empower individuals to make informed decisions about their care. Learning about available treatments, self-care practices, and lifestyle modifications can provide a sense of control and help individuals actively manage their condition.

2. Emotional Support: Building a support network of understanding family members, friends, or support groups can provide emotional support and a sense of community. Sharing experiences, concerns, and coping

strategies with others who have similar experiences can alleviate feelings of isolation and provide valuable insights and encouragement.

3. Self-Care Practices: Engaging in self-care practices can help individuals manage stress, reduce symptoms, and improve overall well-being. This can include activities such as practicing mindfulness and relaxation techniques, pursuing hobbies, engaging in regular exercise, and prioritizing self-care routines that promote

physical and emotional health.

4. Stress Management: Managing stress is crucial in coping with the challenges of LS. Stress can exacerbate symptoms and negatively impact psychological well-being. Implementing stress management techniques such as deep breathing exercises, meditation, yoga, or seeking professional help, such as counseling or therapy, can assist individuals in managing stress and enhancing coping skills.

5. Pain Management: Developing strategies to manage pain associated with LS can improve overall quality of life. This may involve working closely with healthcare providers to identify appropriate pain management techniques, such as topical or oral analgesics, heat or cold therapy, or alternative therapies like acupuncture or physical therapy.

6. Healthy Lifestyle Choices: Maintaining a healthy lifestyle can support overall well-being and help manage LS symptoms. This

includes eating a balanced diet, staying hydrated, getting regular exercise, avoiding potential triggers or irritants, and managing comorbidities such as obesity, diabetes, or autoimmune conditions that may worsen LS symptoms.

7. Seeking Professional Help: Consulting with healthcare professionals who specialize in LS, such as dermatologists, gynecologists, or urologists, is essential for accurate diagnosis, treatment guidance, and ongoing care. They can provide personalized

treatment plans, monitor disease progression, and address specific concerns related to LS.

8. Psychological Support: Seeking psychological support from therapists, counselors, or psychologists experienced in working with chronic conditions can be beneficial. They can help individuals navigate the emotional impact of LS, manage anxiety or depression, and develop coping strategies to enhance overall well-being.

9. Patient Advocacy Organizations: Connecting with patient advocacy organizations specializing in LS can provide valuable resources, information, and support. These organizations often offer educational materials, online communities, and opportunities for individuals to engage in advocacy efforts or participate in research studies.

10. Regular Follow-up Care: Regular follow-up care with healthcare providers is essential to monitor the progression of

LS, adjust treatment plans if necessary, and address any new symptoms or concerns. This helps ensure that individuals receive ongoing support, stay informed about advancements in treatment options, and have access to appropriate care.

Coping with LS is a personal journey, and individuals may find that different strategies work best for them at different times. It is important to be patient with oneself, practice self-compassion, and seek support when needed. By utilizing coping strategies, accessing support networks, and engaging in self-care, individuals with LS can navigate the challenges associated with the condition and improve their overall quality of life and psychological well-being.

www.ingramcontent.com/pod-product-compliance
Lightning Source LLC
Chambersburg PA
CBHW051822250726
48659CB00005B/1622